Fresh
Squeezed

Toni

You matter!

Love,

Fresh Squeezed

A COSTA RICAN JOURNEY OF FASTING AND SELF-DISCOVERY

• • •

written by

Phyllis Adler, LCSW–R

illustrated by Marlin Peterson • *edited by* Cat Thomson

Fresh Squeezed: A Costa Rican Journey of Fasting and Self-Discovery
Copyright © 2014 by Phyllis Adler

Author photo by Phyllis Adler
Book design by Emma Schlieder
Illustrations by Marlin Peterson

Printed in the United States of America

The Troy Book Makers • Troy, New York • thetroybookmakers.com

To order additional copies of this title, contact your favorite local bookstore or visit www.tbmbooks.com

ISBN: 978-1-61468-230-1

Acknowledgements

. . . .

I want to thank the following people:

To Cat — thank you for your remarkable, steadfast, caring, and thoughtful approach to this project.

To Marlin — you took words and brought them to life. Thank you for your vision and talents.

To Matt Smith — thank you for the brainstorming time and coming up with the title!

To my dear friend Janet — Your support, love, and friendship is like a good cup of Caribou coffee. Hugs to you.

To Judy and Jim — thank you for taking me into your heart as one of your own.

To my college friends who know their importance in my life — lest I leave someone out — thank you for loving me every day even as distance separates us.

To my high school teachers — you filled me up enough to get me through. Thank you for your hugs.

To my friends here at home — your patience with my ever changing perspective is appreciated.

To Joanne S. — I won't ever forget your life saving words…"can you believe in my belief in you" until I could find my own…

To my siblings — thank you for your support and love.

To my nephew Kevin — your very existence gives me joy. I love you "that big" now and always.

To Karen — thank you for being my base.

To the Capital District YMCA — your facilities offered me (and still do) a place where my mind and body work themselves out.

To my aunt Fran — thank you for your unrelenting support, encouragement, wisdom, and initial editing of this book. This project could *only* be done with YOU. [The basics of this book were written during a winter storm in NYC in Fran's apartment. Thereafter, Fran would take the train early in the morning from NYC to Albany where we would work on the book at the Amtrak station, and then return late afternoon. She took this trip every Sunday until the project was completed.] Fran, thank you for those hours on the train, and all you sacrificed to do that. And thank you for coming into my life.

To Katherine Croll and your Gentle Earth Retreat — without you, this project would never have existed. I thank you for all it inspired. I thank you for helping to heal my mind, body, and soul…for without health, the other two could not thrive. You gave me hope back in Ithaca when I first took a sip — thank you.

This book is dedicated to Brendan Parnell, a fellow juicer I met the following year at Gentle Earth Retreat. His life ended much too soon, but his quest will never be forgotten and may be best understood through his music. The guitar he traveled with was dusty and unused for some time before his arrival but on day four, he took it out of its case and began to play. May your family take comfort in knowing you touched so many lives.

Introduction

· ·

Here, begins my quest: The Juice Fast.

Location: Gentle Earth Retreat, Costa Rica

Time frame: 10 days

In retrospect, a childhood of fear.

A single mother, ruthlessly abusive. An absent father. Haunting memories of threadbare shoes, wearing the same set of clothing for days at a time, and subsisting on the pasty taste of government cheese, powdered milk, and rice and beans.

My newly acquired adult years were punctuated by a simple surgery gone awry coupled with an incapacitating bike riding accident, each exacerbating my already diagnosed inability to poop.

Surprise! All of this was accompanied by an obsession with food.

All roads lead to the JUICE FAST.

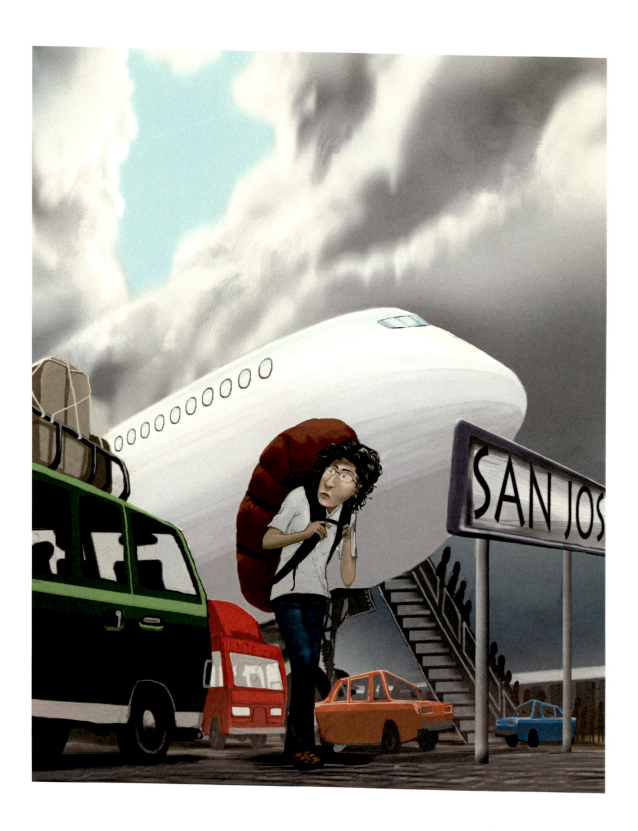

Those who say 'half the fun is getting there' have never traveled

One backpack full of basics: a pair of shorts, a few tops, hybrid shoes, and a diary.

Having left behind a heavy load of digestive aids, my anxiety ridden body finds its way into a scheduled four a.m. taxi. My itinerary is overwhelming. Three plane changes minus the necessary pre-printed boarding passes to confirm my flights.

I arrive at Albany International at four-thirty in the morning only to find that it's an intimate encounter between me and the security guard, as the airport does not officially open until five. At the enchanted hour, showing my passport to the guard, I am directed downstairs to a ticket agent. There, I am pointed to the self-serve kiosk. Sir, I need an agent! As fellow early bird desperados take up the cry, the ticket agent now outnumbered, motions 'come hither to the counter,' thus beginning the singing tone of passes being printed.

Tenacity! Leg one – completed.

Arrival, airport – Dulles International. Now looking for TACA airlines, I use my once in another lifetime, six mile-a-day running legs to follow the maze of signs leading to a bus that leads to the tram that leads to the Spanish only signs of TACA. Reading my itinerary for the twelfth time (I have never been accused of being obsessive compulsive), I secure my next boarding pass. Seat 12D. Off to San Salvador, El Salvador.

Oh my G-d! The pilot's announcements are in Spanish. Before I can stage a meltdown, however, the announcements begin again, this time in English.

At two in the afternoon, my ears rhythmically popping from the altitude, I hastily begin to practice my deep breathing. I hit the alert button. The summoned stewardess continues to smile throughout my hysterical rant pertaining to my soon to be missed two-fifteen connection from El Salvador to Costa Rica. How is it that the entire plane knew, even the gurgling infant two aisles down, that my watch needed to be turned back by one hour? It was only one in the afternoon in Central America.

Landed. A sign points to the *bano*. Ugh. San Salvador bathrooms expect you to wipe and throw the toilet paper in garbage cans. Double Ugh! Not sure why, but there is no time to ask about that particular law of the land, as I am gathering my fortitude to make that third connection!

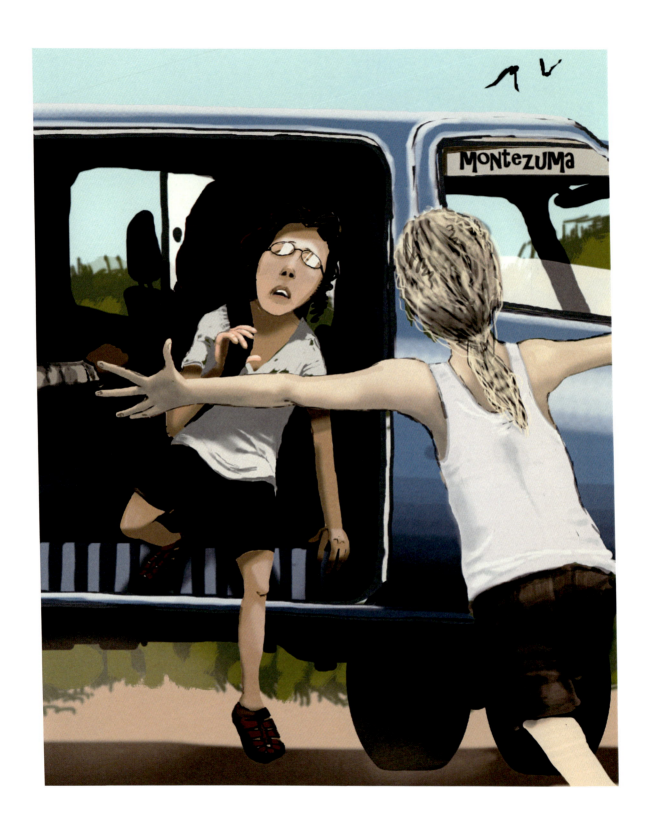

Connection made. Landing in Costa Rica, another maze, this one of immigration lines. My passport now stamped, I find myself outdoors waving paperwork in an attempt to attract anyone speaking English. Among the crowd of taxi drivers steps forward my own personal Don Quixote minus the sword. We speed off to my booked hotel.

Morning. The ride. It is a van from Montezuma Expeditions, the entity that has arranged my travel throughout this trip to Costa Rica. (A more appropriate name would Montezuma's Revenge.) My head is getting a workout. Through tumbling rocks and dirt paths that can barely fit a full size car, let alone this van, the road slowly inclines to vertical and like all things that go up, well, the road eventually must come down. As I slide into the other passengers that are to my left and then those that are to my right, ditches catch the wheels and without struts or shocks, this van becomes my object of prayer. As my head hits the roof — again, there appears a never ending cycle of mountain terrain and volcanic smoke that gravitate "aaahhh" from my fellow travelers, but not from me. I am sweaty. I cross my legs. I have to pee. I now cannot think of anything else but the time. Two in the afternoon. Again? Oh no — that was yesterday.

A century later, passing orange, green, and yellow bungalows, my driver makes a right and stops abruptly (there goes my head again) at a wooden fence. Is he lost? Will I just be left here! Racing thoughts — I never even asked the driver if he knew where he was taking me. First that two hour ferry ride and now this three hour drive to…? My silent expletives race even faster, I look up.

A wooden gate slides open and she appears. Big smile, blonde hair, long with some stray curls. She stands tall and clean. Having not showered in days, my newly formed grey hairs grease over my glasses and my knapsack clings to my t-shirt. Reunion — it's Katherine from New York. Her arms open wide as I scrunch my way out of the van. A hug. Gladly accepted. A weary smile forms on my lips as I mouth the words, "juice fast needed, very badly."

LESSONS LEARNED

- Learn Spanish – at least a little bit. **Bano** means bathroom. That word is good to know in any language.

- Pack gum to combat the effects of flying at a high altitude.

- Above all, this is a lesson in **paciencia** – patience. Enjoy the bumps as your journey will test your determination and perseverance. Take it one step at a time. If you don't have patience it is guaranteed that something will happen to remind you that you need it.

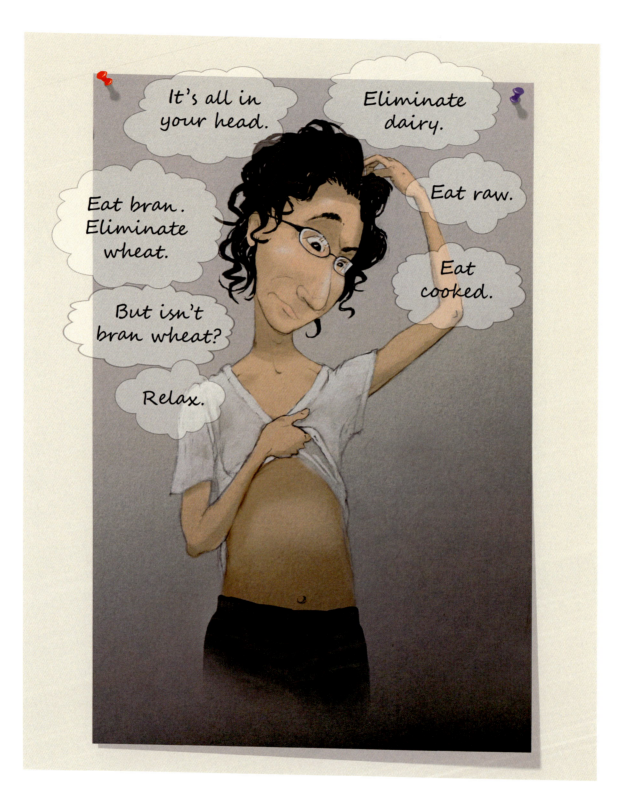

Hallmark might disagree that 'Home is where the juice is'

Conflicting advice from family, friends, and doctors. Eat raw. Eat cooked. Eat more frequently. Eat less frequently. Have fruit. No, have vegetables. Eliminate dairy – but kefir is dairy! Eat bran. Eliminate wheat. But isn't bran wheat? Oh, I so wish I could just eliminate. Try yoga. Relax. It's all in your head. Yes, that's right. All of these contradictions are reeling in my head.

Nine in the morning, Costa Rica time.

The menu on the whiteboard has six entrees:

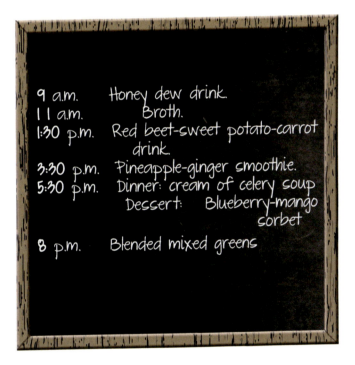

9 a.m.   Honey dew drink.
11 a.m.   Broth.
1:30 p.m. Red beet-sweet potato-carrot drink.
3:30 p.m. Pineapple-ginger smoothie.
5:30 p.m. Dinner: cream of celery soup
           Dessert: Blueberry-mango sorbet

8 p.m.   Blended mixed greens

The Juice Fast has begun.

What's the attraction? It is believed by those who have successfully juiced that the immune system is centered around the gut, which is comprised of the stomach and intestines. As a result, juicers believe that many illnesses stem from problems in this area. When juicing, the digestive process is essentially placed on hold so that the immune system can work on other areas of the body that are in need of attention.

During a juice fast, we drink. We drink *a lot*. For every drink on the menu, we must intake eight ounces of water; this is in addition to a daily detox tea of our choice and a green tea. A part of the juice fast requires getting acquainted, between the morning drink and broth time, with a handy dandy 32 oz. enema bag. A coffee enema brewed daily is gracefully offered to me. For the newbie, Katherine is there to teach the art of the enema. And then, we are good to go.

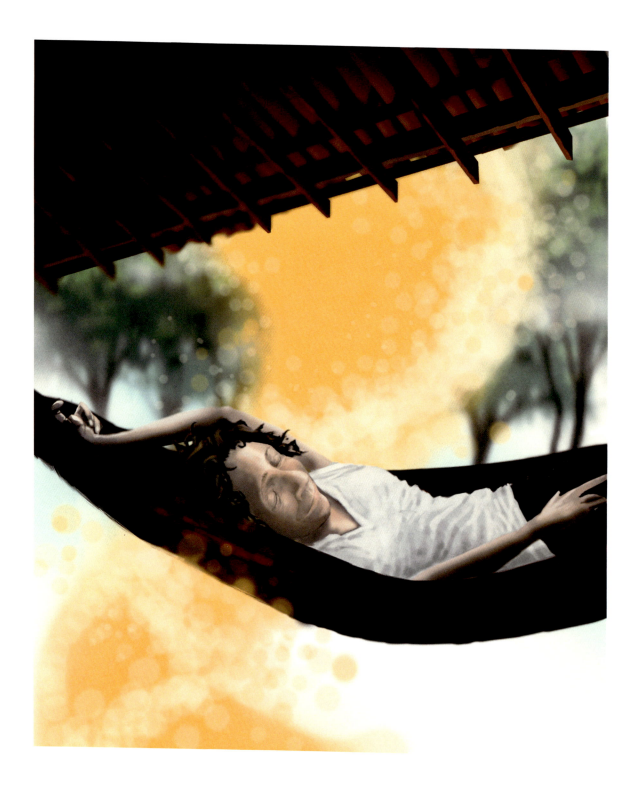

Here, where the juice fast takes place, I am home. The patio off the main house has been artistically tiled by Katherine. It becomes my outdoor abode for many of the daily rituals of juicing. Its pathway leads to the entrance of a lush rain forest and animal life mecca. It is here that geckos, roosters, and horses share the land, collectively calling it their own. Hammocks invite relaxation.

I drink. I pee. I cry. I smile. I am childlike as I joke about almost pooping in my pants. I play with Pedro, Katherine's Chihuahua. As a child, I imagined galloping on a horse using my fingers on the kitchen table – an escape? I remember wanting to be a cowgirl and would cut out one dimensional ads of ranch hands galloping on horseback. Here, I dance next to a farm horse, swaying side to side.

Now there is space between my feelings and my thoughts. My breathing begins to mimic the calmness of my surroundings as I experience a quiet redemption. Although at first it eludes articulation, I am wiser, sitting studiously with my diary at poolside. I begin writing feverishly.

Done for the day, I make my way past bungalows that are covered in plumage of rich yellows, greens, and orange. In my room, the painting of a swan on the ceramic wall does little to hide the iguana that is hanging from the ceiling. In the middle of the night at Gentle Earth Retreat, I hear monkeys that sound like lions roaring. I dream in colors of ginger, coconut, and mango.

LESSONS LEARNED

- Know where the bathrooms are as they will come in handy, especially when wearing good clothing.

- A journey to an unfamiliar physical location may actually afford an opportunity to relax and let one's guard down. It may prove to be what is necessary to begin to confront the past, accept it, and make plans to move on.

- Juicing may allow for introspection as the body is not focused on breaking down what has been ingested.

- Why be satisfied with merely surviving when thriving is in reach?

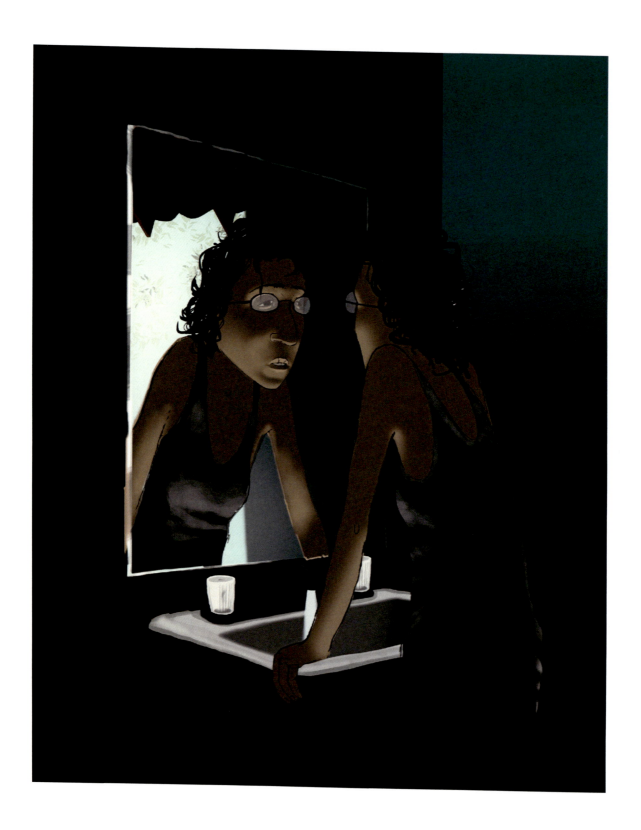

Oh, Those Simple Words

Jason, now eight pounds lighter from juicing, carries a dog-eared book under his arm while balancing a cup of detox tea in one hand and his red drink in the other. Arriving a few days earlier than I, he was just in time to experience the end of Costa Rica's rainy season – a mudslide and rock avalanche.

We are now both poolside. I have transitioned from Keens all terrain shoes into flip flops and staged my chair so that I may take in the afternoon sun. Reclining, eyes closed, I find myself cycling in and out of thoughts that in the very recent past verged on an obsessive pattern of fears, pain, and sadness. I grieve silently. Today, however, there is an assemblage of clarity, perhaps due to the amino acids from my afternoon juicing.

Jason, sensing my inner struggle, whispers, "I need do nothing" as he points to these exact words in his book. This simple sentence "I need do nothing" spoken ever so soothingly, incredibly, allows me to stop seeking control over what cannot be changed and relax, at least for the moment.

My mind is now focused. I reflect on what I am grateful for: high school teachers, the bagel store job that as a teenager became my refuge, college friends, counselors, and more currently, Katherine's Juice Fast that is bringing me closer to good health.

As others have helped me, I, as a social worker, now provide therapy to troubled families. In the past, I was given. I now give.

LESSONS LEARNED

- Learn to juggle. The art of balancing is needed in life.

- Take the time to appreciate the individuals you have encountered, who have made a difference with their presence.

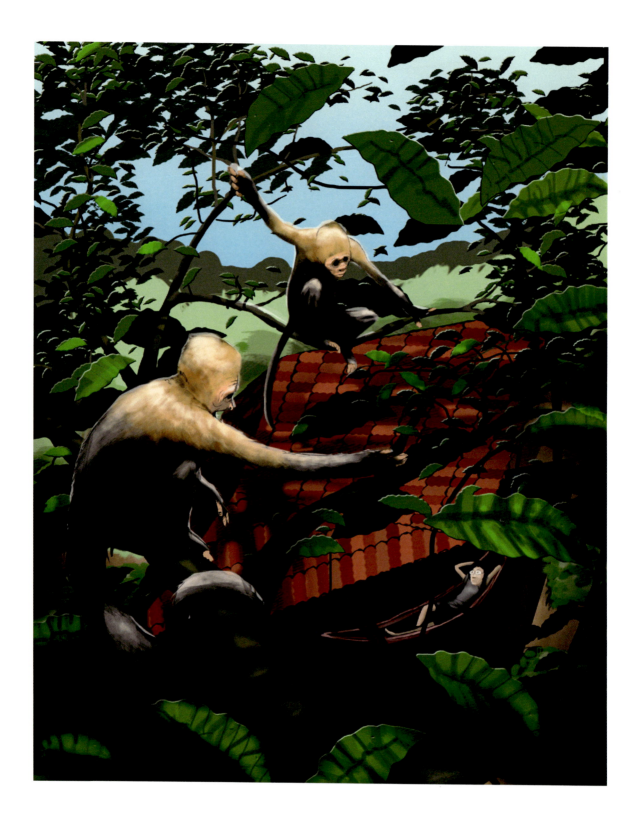

Night Night (Bananas Not Included)

The sun sets and night time is upon us. Las Vegas? Not quite. Loud? Yes. At intervals, the trees come alive with the sound of music from little white faced monkeys. They are known in the quaint village of Cabuya as the howler monkeys. Their cry is a cross between a lion's roar and a horse's neigh. Their volley of conversation sounds quite serious from my open bedroom window. These sounds, for no explicable reason, trigger the funny bone inside me. I giggle to myself and realize that I am out-sounded.

For the moment, I prefer these tones to the beeping of cars, the sounds of bustling computer keys, managers speaking in high pitched tones, and the ongoing battle with many of my co-workers regarding a high versus a low thermostat setting.

The guttural sounds of these small-faced primates brings out the child in me. As I mimic their speech, "eeeeaaaahhhhuuuuuu" I am one with these monkeys! Having had no idea I had this in me, my cry becomes louder and louder and is heard by my juicing companions. My two buddies begin to make sounds of their own. Christine imitates a rooster's call and Jason does the whinny of a horse. I was told that on day four of the juice fast, the body may experience euphoria. For this trio, it has manifested into unabashed laughter.

LESSONS LEARNED

- Have fun. Let the monkey out! It will go a long way in repairing damage that has been done.

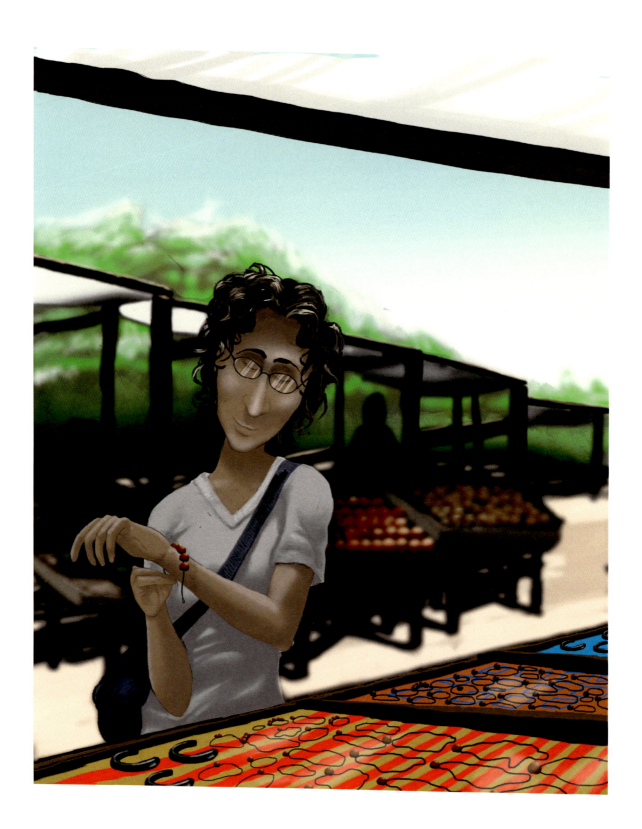

Axles Are Essential

Departure by bus, two-fifteen in the afternoon. Pickup is where the path to Katherine's house ends. Villagers assemble.

We Wait. Two-thirty.

Katherine and I are scheduled to take a stroll through Montezuma (all one strip mall-like block of it) where the ocean is a hand's breadth away. She has packed "Cas," a drink made from an exotic fruit tasting somewhat like a cross between applesauce and peach. When it is poured and my tongue meets the glass, it is like a reunion of two lost souls.

We wait. She confidently hands me *colones* to pay for boarding the bus.

We wait.

Katherine at last inquires in half Spanish and half hand gesture. She is told the bus's axle may not have been repaired.

"Let's start walking," Katherine suggests. "Not sure if the bus is coming," she concludes.

"Seven miles. Each way? Only one bus?" Walk using my feet? New York City – not.

I am dumbfounded. My need is to be in control. What happened to *the* plan? Katherine is nonchalant and accepting of an alternative that will allow us to safely hitch-hike if our feet give out. With Katherine's urging, my hybrid shoes begin to apprehensively put one foot in front of the other. To my amazement, a driver swings by in his four wheeler. We are offered a ride.

The driver stops. We arrive at our destination, the center of the town of Montezuma. Languages spoken in the street range from Australian style English to Dutch. The beach front is sandy and invites a swim. The colors of the storefronts remind me of old western movies. As Katherine escorts me around, I stay on her arm like a little kid-soaking it all in. The locals are friendly and willing to chat. I fall in love with a handmade coconut bracelet that I purchase.

We walk. It is work. Uphill and downhill. Road-like. Within me, there is now a need to redefine my definition of work, and with it that of life itself.

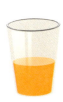

LESSONS LEARNED

- Know people with cars. Better yet, know a good mechanic.

- Do not turn back. Be flexible. It will get you where you need to go.

- Re-examine your options.

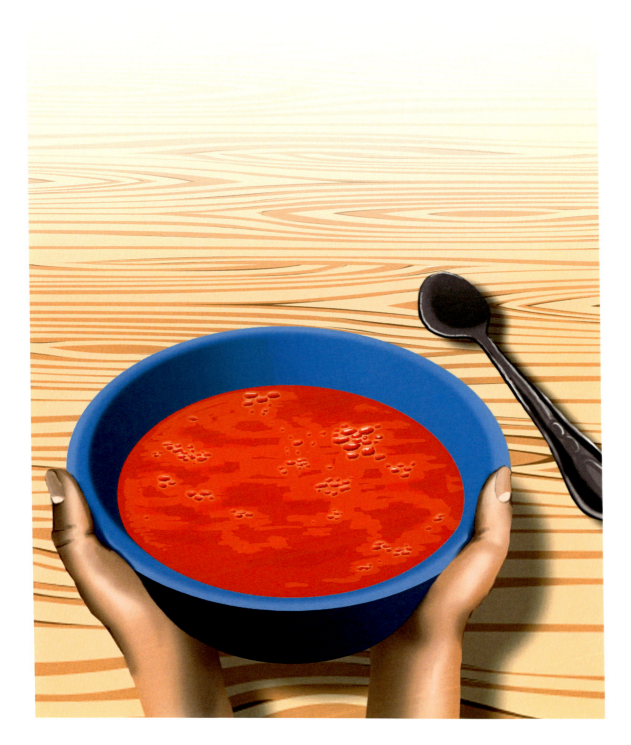

The Art of the Soup Bowl

Here I sit. Eighty degrees. Dinner time.

The strung patio lights are reminiscent of Rockefeller Center during the winter holiday season.

A menu of soups already experienced by juicing – carrot-ginger, cream of spinach, mushroom, and cream of celery. Tonight, it's red-pepper.

Slurp from the bowl? My hands are drawn to its ceramic surface. Do I dare? Aside from possible embarrassment due to a breach in etiquette, what is the worst scenario? Will I be given a time out? Dismissed from the table and barred from coming back? Will Katherine yell in Seinfeld fashion "NO SOUP FOR YOU!"?

I momentarily grapple with and then forgo all Western convention and bring the bowl to my lips with newfound courage and gusto. My eyes catch the bulging stares from my dinner mates. I offer no excuses but merely a simple statement, "I hope you don't mind, I'm drinking from the bowl."

"I have been wanting to do that," Jason states as he and Christine, to my amazement, follow my lead.

Katherine and her husband, Jeff, act as our surrogate parents. "You may drink from your bowl, but not too fast. It's bad for digestion and one needs to appreciate the aroma and flavor."

We three nod in agreement.

LESSONS LEARNED

- Etiquette, smediquette. When you believe in a cause worth fighting for- if need be, stand alone. Take your time. Savor— *deliciosa.*

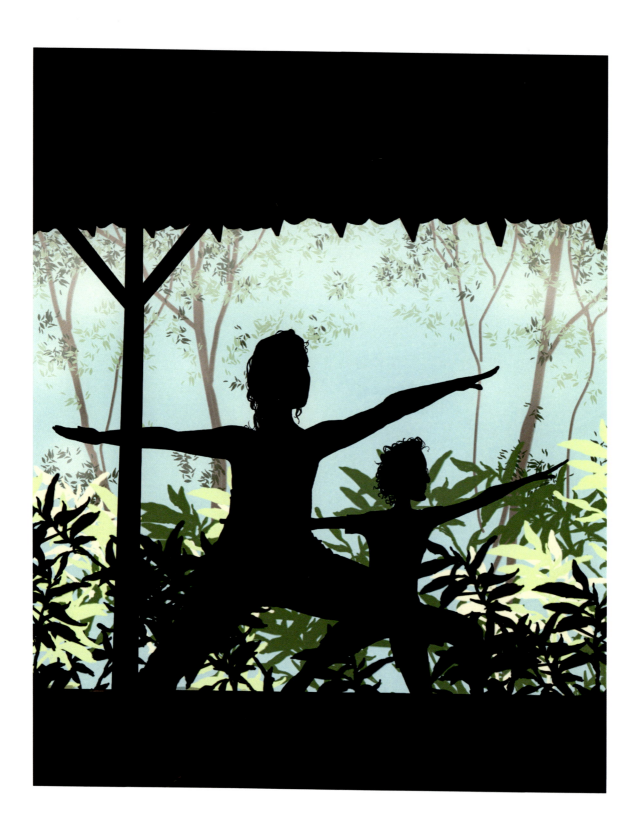

Breathing required—although that does not make for proficient relaxation

Eleven-thirty am. I am in a yoga move. Again.

Breathing in. Breathing out. My life is one breath. My mind, on the other hand, is fixated on the past and future. I don't really love the east coast cold. I am nervous to leave what now feels like home.

I see the sweat pouring off Jason. Arms widen. Airplane move. Lift off, chest up, legs raised off the ground. This is ridiculous.

Next move. I am prepared – I have memorized them. Tree move. Warrior move. No wonder they call it warrior – I am now staring meanly for no reason whatsoever – because it is called warrior? Why don't I just do a lunge. Essentially, that's the move. I twist my head left and my left arm reaches to the imaginary "nothingness" that I am now commanded to focus on. All the while keeping as steady as a shocked deer caught in a headlights. Hold it. DON'T MOVE!

(Urge to cough. Urge to drink. Urge to find Pedro. Urge to call my sister and my aunt. Urge to pee. Urge to poop? Not yet.)

Urges distract me from this outdoor exercise. Determined to fully embrace and understand any possible benefit this could have for me, I say hello to my feet again. Abs. Slowly I raise my upper body, twisting left and then right, all the while pretending as instructed that I have a ball in my hands. I don't get it.

I am, however, strangely drawn to attempt to understand the resistance inside me. My fellow juicers are so into this! I want my one-twenty p.m. drink.

Focus. At the usual twelve-thirty time, I am instructed to breathe and just listen to the gentle rings of both the bells and meditation bowls. I can do THAT!

I understand. I fall into that calming place within my mind. Hands at my side. I feel a rush as I let go. I am guided into allowing my thoughts to dissipate into a picture of the sun's rays entering my head and following the trail to my feet. Done. Without force, I agree to come back tomorrow.

LESSONS LEARNED

- Try something that exercises both the physical and mental. Yoga? Maybe. Maybe not. Results may not be immediate. Try, try, try again. Due to my exposure to yoga, I find myself breathing in a manner that is calming, particularly around my hyper-caffeinated co-workers. It may be worth hanging in there for a bit longer, especially if the guidance you get comes from someone who is a happy warrior.

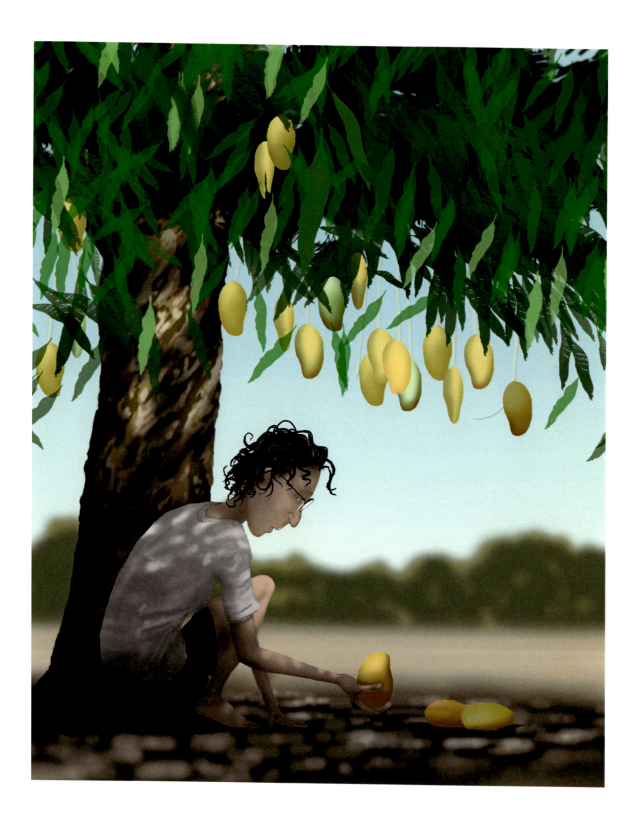

Falling hurts, even at your own pace

Alone. I am walking in Cabuya. I have come to love this little village. Mind you, my eleven a.m. ritual drink of sweet potato-carrot-beet sets me up for loving most anything. There is something special in the air here. With my newly formed language skills, which incorporate a bit of creative license, I can now communicate quite confidently with some of the more patient villagers.

I imagine living here.

Mango trees are everywhere. Mangos are pretty. They are big and mushy. They taste great in smoothies. Mango-blueberry, mango-starfruit… My mango. My love.

In my desperate desire to savor the moment, I sit and study its texture. What made this one fall? Was it ripe? Was it the wind?

In my now drunkard demeanor that blubbers love of this planet, I look up to the home of the mango. Piercing the sky's rays, I call out, "Why and when did you fall?" The mango, thankfully, does not answer. I am now Tom Hanks with his volleyball, shipwrecked on an island as I remember him in "Cast Away."

Falling is never easy even when you can lessen the impact by knowing how to break the fall. I sit with them - *los mangos*.

LESSONS LEARNED

- Keep your hands clean. You never know when you have to use them for talking.

- It is okay to sit on the ground and examine things.

- Like mangos we fall. It may be anticipated or totally unexpected. Accept that it has happened. There is a reason. You may be severely bruised. Remember, your essence has not changed. After all, the mango is still the mango.

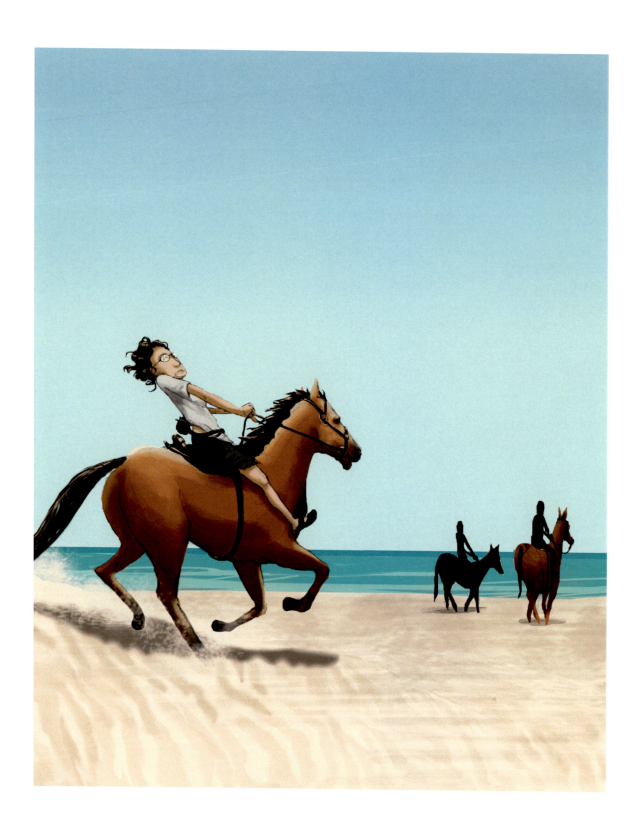

Horses do speak, but not in English

I am face to face with my mode of transportation for a sightseeing expedition. The HORSE. No Marlboro magazine pictures – this is the real deal.

I nod to my guide as I learn that he does not speak English, and my ego must now admit that my Spanish is oh so limited. With a stiff upper lip (I admit it was quivering), my amateur status as a horseback rider is evidenced by my hesitancy in mounting onto the saddle.

Christine and another traveler hop on and, in unison, flag the guide with waving hands that I, Phyllis, am not at all familiar with this horse thing. The guide, in return, gives a short pantomime lesson of "pull toward you to stop, to the left and to the right" for the obvious. We are off – to the waterfall that we signed up to see – one and a half hours each way.

Time now, two pm. What's with me and this two pm hour???

Clinging to the reigns, trotting over twigs, fallen branches and trees, amidst rock pilings, I come to appreciate the concept of butt on saddle coordination. I'm honest. I have none. "Squeeze your thighs!" yells Christine, seeing my perplexed mouth now open in fright. Squeeze my thighs? Where? I squeeze against the horse. My butt hurts. My spine hurts. I bounce up and down hitting the saddle hard. Up and down, up and down… This is not working. I begin to talk to my horse. He has no clue.

Now the climb. I didn't know there was a climb! The sign for horseback riding did not say climb. Climb indicates vertical. VERTICAL. I cannot turn back. My guide and my companions are well ahead of me. I yell but I am not heard. I breathe. Does the horse know not to walk soooo close to the edge of the cliff? My legs get tangled in low hanging tree limbs. With patience and my horse's cooperation, I break free. Catching up to my comrades, one is now positioned in front of me, the other remains in back. Climbing, I am instructed to lean forward and lift myself off the stirrups. Going down, I lean back. This I get.

Reaching the sandy beach, which was advertised, I once again try not to give in to panic and begin my breathing exercise as my horse's cantor turns into an unrehearsed gallop. Ouch, ouch, ouch. Back and ribs are jostled. Butt on saddle. Thighs not squeezing. I pull the reigns. Horse slows down. Horse speeds up. I pull again. I cannot do the gallop. Christine tells me that my horse is young and childlike. "He wants to run so you have to keep reminding him to slow down." Horse like a child. My horse is in control – I am not. I now pull and pull again and again. To my wonderment, my heart is still beating. Finally. The waterfall.

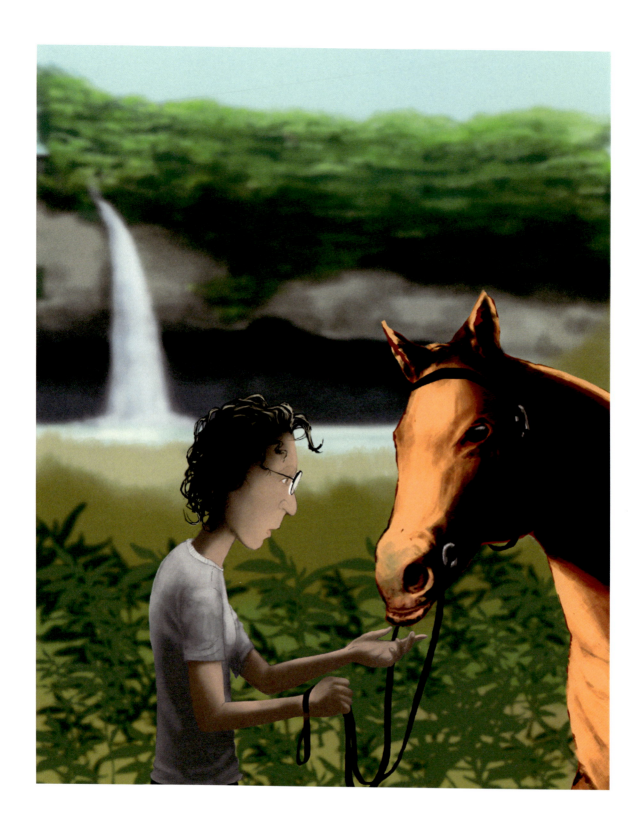

We dismount and our guide ties up the horses to a tree. We walk up a rock and, out of a bag, our guide pulls out a pineapple. Christine and I motion that we decline - juice fast. I point to the precious drinks that I was assigned to carry and have since spilled due to my inexperience as a rider. David, the third rider, accepts. My guide takes his machete from his waistband. Delicately and with precision, he slices the skin off the pineapple and makes little servings for himself and David. Yum. My tongue reaches out and then back in. I admonish myself silently. No breaking the juice fast.

We admire the waterfall - the highlight of the ride.

Riding back, I practice the art of coordination. Rise up and keep those thighs squeezed. When properly galloping, the butt and saddle become one. What a wonderful feeling! A sense of accomplishment. My ride back is almost flawless. No pulling — a near perfect rhythm when galloping. I am in control and the horse and I now speak to each other in a language we can both understand.

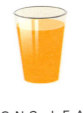

LESSONS LEARNED

- Have a chiropractor's number.

- When packing juice, tighten the lid a few extra times. Triple check.

- Once again, breathing properly comes in handy.

- Horses can be intimidating as can any means to a desired end. We have the ability to do what needs to be done. Fears will pass. Coordination of both the mind and body will happen. It will all come together. Do not give up.

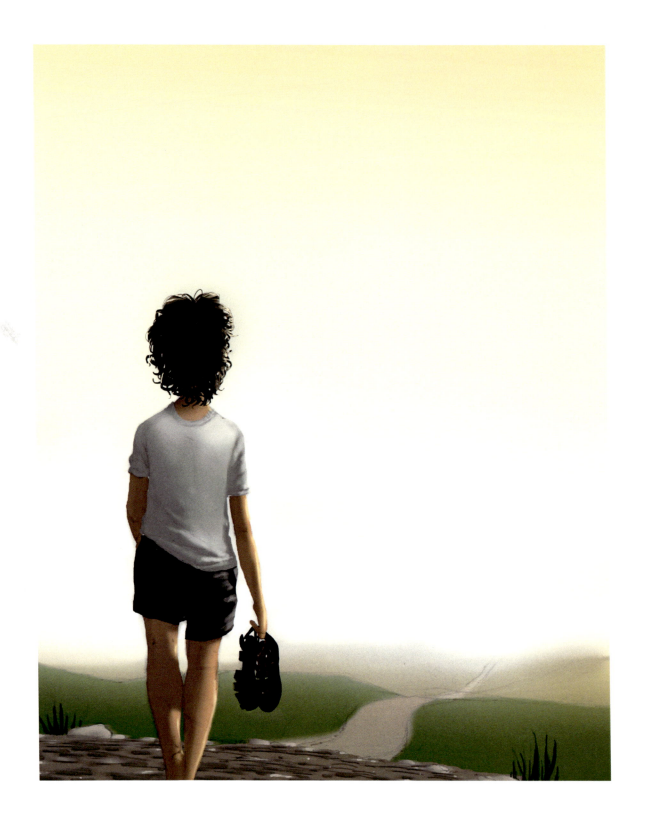

It's all in the Dirt

Dirt. My last day. Dirt. I will even miss the dirt here. It has exhaust-like smells from the ATV's and mopeds that race by. My throat is scratchy. The dirt in the potholes has small particles of rock. My shoes are now covered in dust and I walk in mindful meditation. The juicing is over. I tearfully stare into the dirt. I heed the yoga instruction – *Namaste* – appreciate, be present.

Saying goodbye is not easy. My face feels smooth and my insides have no pain. My body is lean and my mind is aware.

This juice fast in Costa Rica, in the village of Cabuya, has inspired me to set goals. I can think clearly. I have learned that food cannot compensate for time lost.

My work back home will continue to address the parental love that was absconded in my childhood and the voice that I was denied. As a therapist to others, I will pass on the acronym L.O.V.E. – Listen, Observe, Validate, Encourage – which this juice fast has given me the liberty to devise.

Ten days in Costa Rica.

LESSONS LEARNED

- Bring hybrid shoes for walking.

- Eye shadow is totally unnecessary.

- Pack two diaries. Write, write, and write.

- Find your quest. It's your journey.

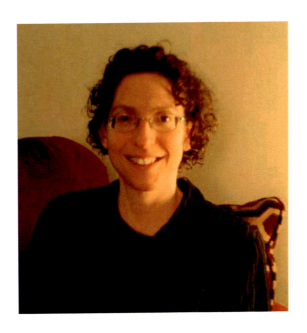

Phyllis Adler, LCSW-R is a Licensed Clinical Social Worker, and has spent over 16 years providing counseling to children, youth, and families. Her specialty is child abuse. She is Founder of Counseling Sense and a member of Prevent Child Abuse NY. Her framework of L.O.V.E. (Listen, Observe, Validate, Encourage) was developed while on her juice fast and she now educates others on the topics of resilience, trauma, healing, and therapy. Whether the issue is addiction, self-esteem, or abuse, Phyllis captures the heart of the matter and creates an atmosphere for growth. Raised in New York City, Phyllis is one of five children who survived poverty and abuse. Despite having never played a single game on the high school basketball team for which she was manager, she was awarded the MVP, a symbol of the leadership she embodies. Though trials continued, her journey ultimately led to the juice fast at Gentle Earth Retreat, a place that now serves as her once-a-year refuge and where she calls "home." She can be contacted at **counselingsense@yahoo.com** or you can check out her website at **www.counselingsense.com.**

• • •